CW00862738

Skinny is Be:

A combination of fast weight loss diets, food

plans, exercise and more

by

Denise James

Published by Skinny is Best Publication

Cover design created by Denise James

Disclaimer Notice

This book is designed to provide information on weight loss, diets, and fitness exercise only. This information is provided and sold with the knowledge that the publisher and author do not offer any legal or other professional advice. In the case of a need for any such expertise consult with the appropriate professional. This book does not contain all information available on the subject. This book has not been created to be specific to any individual's or organisation's situation or needs. Every effort has been made to make this book as accurate as possible. However, there may be typographical and or content errors. Therefore, this book should serve only as a general guide and not as the ultimate source of subject information. This book contains information that might be dated and is intended only to educate and entertain. The author and publisher shall have no liability or responsibility to any person or entity regarding any loss or damage incurred, or alleged to have incurred, directly or indirectly, by the information contained in this book. You hereby agree to be bound by this disclaimer.

Introduction

A nonfiction book about fast weight loss dieting, food plans, exercise regimes for a faster working metabolism, helpful tips on herbal teas, and other diets that have been all tried by myself, the author of this book.

This book is written in my own words and is a compilation of articles from My Weight Loss and Diet Life Blog. If you need to lose weight quickly, this book can help you. There are a few ways that you can lose weight faster. Food plans for these diets have been listed in this book.

I have tried all the diet food plans in this book and I can say that they have worked for me and others. Take a look at Skinny is Best website for more information and read the comments of others who have tried *The Chemical Diet*.

Please note: If you have a health problem, please consult with your doctor before trying any kind of diet whether it is from this book or not.

Do You Need to Lose Weight in a Hurry?

Have you ever been in a situation where you had to attend an event and you couldn't find anything you could wear, because you were too overweight? I have.

The answer may be yes if you have decided to read this book or if you have an event to attend and you have left dieting to the last minute. Have you got a wedding to go to or a planned holiday that is coming up sooner than you thought? Sometimes, we get into a panic about our weight, because an outfit will not fit us in time for that big party. I know I have been in situations like this before. It's a horrible feeling

8

and I hate it. No doubt, you must hate it too!

I had this idea that most people must feel this way whenever they are about to attend something important in their lives and we want to be able to look good for it.

Well, if that is the case, then read on and find out what you can do to lose weight quickly and then continue it for a healthy weight loss regime.

This book will help you decide very quickly on what to do about your weight loss goals if you are stuck on what to do. There is a special one-week diet that can help you lose up to one stone in this book and that's *The Chemical Diet.*

Table of Contents

13

1. The Chemical Diet Where You Can Lose a Stone in One Week

The Chemical Diet has been around for years, but have you ever heard of it? Not many people have really. James Duncan wrote about this diet and tried it himself. I have now tried it a number of times. It's one of those diets that can come in handy if you need to lose a few pounds before an event you are attending or even if you have decided to go on holiday at the last minute.

The Chemical Diet is for people who need to lose weight before surgery or for anyone that needs to shift weight quickly. You do the diet for one week every three weeks. I tried this diet and it helped me to lose weight. The only drawback is that you have to stick to this diet food plan.

The Chemical Diet is a 7-day food plan that you stick to every three weeks. Apparently, from what I have heard from others, you can lose one stone by just sticking to the exact food plan that I have included below. Can you believe that it can work? I wasn't sure about it at first, but when I tried it, after two days I could see the weight fall away from me.

It truly does work. I tried it and lost nearly a stone. Anyone can do it.

The following is the food plan that was

recommended by James Duncan, where he writes on how he lost a stone doing the Chemical Diet. You can, also, read the comments on his blog below on how others have tried the diet and lost weight.

Click here: The Chemical Diet

Here is the food plan for one week:

Day	Breakfast	Lunch	Dinner
1	1 slice dry toast with 1 grilled fresh tomato or tinned tomatoes	Fresh fruit - any amount	2-hard boiled eggs Salad 1 grapefruit
2	1 Grapefruit 1 boiled egg	Grilled or roast chicken (any amount) with 2 large	Grilled steak Salad

		fresh tomatoes Toast	
3	Grapefruit 1 boiled egg	Fresh fruit - any amount	2 grilled lamb chops Salad 1 grapefruit
4	1 slice of dry toast	Fresh fruit - any amount	2 boiled hard eggs salad
5	1 slice of dry toast	Fresh fruit - any amount	Fresh fish Salad
6	1 glass grapefruit	Fresh fruit - any amount	Grilled chicken

	juice		Carrots
			1 grapefruit
7	2 Scrambled eggs 1-large grilled tomato	2 poached eggs Spinach	Grilled steak Salad

Note:

Do not eat anything that is not mentioned.

Eat only what is shown or do without.

No substitutions are allowed.

No eating between meals.

No alcohol.

No butter milk or fat.

Drinks = black tea, black coffee, lemon tea, grapefruit juice, tonic, soda, or water only

Salad = lettuce, cucumber, tomatoes, and celery only

DO NOT DIET FOR MORE THAN ONE WEEK AT A TIME.

I recommend the Chemical Diet to anyone that can eat the above food plan for just a week. It's easy if you are determined enough to stick to it and it's a bonus when you start to see the weight fall off. It can, also, start you off on a healthy weight loss journey if you use the Food plan continuously, but add more vegetables, salad, fruit, cottage cheese, and low-fat yogurt to it after the first week. I have done this myself and it does work. You keep on doing the Chemical Diet every third week. Of course, I am not saying it is going to be easy, but after a week on the Chemical Diet, you can be certain that you will have at least lost one stone.

Lately, I have been doing The Chemical Diet every month and it really does the trick and helps you lose a lot of weight quickly. I have managed to keep the weight off too. It's easy once you are in the right frame of mind and you have stuck to the diet for a while. What I normally do is, do the one-week Chemical Diet and then carry on eating the same foods on the meal plan but you can add more vegetables to it along with fat-free cottage cheese. This works and helps you to lose more pounds in those weeks after you have done the Chemical Diet.

weeks after you have done the Chemical Diet.

2. My Result on the Chemical Diet

I did the Chemical Diet and I lost 10 pounds by the end of the week. You can lose up to one stone if you stick to the food plan (which I have listed here).

I found the diet difficult the first three days, but then it got easier on my fourth day. The Chemical Diet can be done quite easily if you put your mind to it and you are serious about losing weight.

On this diet, you are not allowed to have milk in your tea and coffee, but I did have one teaspoon of skimmed milk in my first cup of tea in the mornings and then I had black coffee the rest of the time. Of course, I still lost weight. If I had left out the milk, I would have lost a stone.

On my last day, I ate some grapes, which is not allowed, but I still lost weight.

So, if anyone does this diet and you really need to lose a stone, then they must be strict with themselves and stick to the food plan.

Doing the Chemical Diet is worthwhile if you really need to lose weight quickly, but you must try to continue eating healthily afterward to stop you from putting the pounds back on.

I will do this diet again in three weeks' time to

carry on losing weight. It can benefit anyone that needs to lose a considerable amount of weight and has a target.

3. More Helpful Tips on the Chemical Diet

If you have just realised that you are out of time to lose weight for that big event you have to go to next month, then all is not lost. Just follow the tips below.

There is always something you can do to help you lose weight in a short amount of time. Read on to find out more.

1. Drink green tea or have some Oolong tea or alternate between both. Apparently, it has been known that you can burn 70 additional calories in a 24-hour period by just drinking green tea.

2. Do not drink coffee with milk or sodas full of sugar. Drink water instead. If you must have coffee, then try drinking it black with or without sweetener.

3. Invest in some five-pound weights. Strength training builds lean muscle tissue, which burns more calories - at work or at rest - 24 hours a day, seven days a week. Try doing push-ups or a few squats or lunges. Use the weights to perform simple biceps curls or triceps pulls. Do these exercises three to four times per week and you will see a difference. Strength training can help you burn more fat.

4. Stop having salt on all your food. Salt can cause water retention, making you look and feel bloated. So give it up today!

5. Spice your food up. Apparently, spicing up

your food can raise your metabolism. Eat jalapenos and cayenne peppers, because they can increase your body's release of stress hormones such as adrenaline, which can speed up your metabolism and your ability to burn calories. Eating hot peppers can also reduce your appetite.

6. Do exercise in the evening. Doing exercise in the evening can be beneficial for the body because many people's metabolism sags down toward the end of the day. Go for a thirty-minute walk thirty minutes before dinner. This will raise your metabolic rate which will also keep it elevated for another two or three hours. This will keep you going even after you have stopped moving.

7. Add 20 minutes of exercise each day. Any

exercise will do. If you have an exercise bike or a treadmill at home, then start using it. Lately, I have been doing strength training exercises and I can tell you that doing these exercises have helped me considerably (read no. 3 above).

8. Drink plenty of water every day. It can help. Drink at least two litres per day. It can help with belly fat and if you have water retention.

9. Eat fruit instead of sugary foods.

10. Eat more fish like salmon.

11. Eat boiled eggs for breakfast.

12. If you want to lose weight faster, then read about the Chemical Diet. This is a one-week diet guaranteed to help you lose 14 pounds in that week. Check it out.

13. Cut out bread, but if you have to eat it, then

have wholemeal bread, because it is healthier.

4. The One Week Egg Plan Diet

If you want to lose more than a stone then try the following diet. It has worked for many people who are desperate to lose pounds including myself. It is, also, similar to the Chemical Diet.

The One Week Egg Diet

Day 1

Breakfast- one cup of unsweetened coffee

Lunch- 2 hard-boiled eggs

Dinner- a piece of meat and lemon-based salad

Day 2

Breakfast- one cup of unsweetened coffee and a piece of wholemeal toast dry

Lunch- 2 hard-boiled eggs

Dinner- a piece of ham, salad and one cup of sour cream

Day 3

Breakfast- one cup of unsweetened coffee

Lunch- vegetable and fruit mix

Dinner- 2 hard-boiled eggs, a piece of ham and salad

Day 4

Breakfast- one cup of unsweetened coffee

Lunch- 2 hard-boiled eggs and carrot juice

Dinner- a piece of meat and lemon-based salad

Day 5

Breakfast- grated carrots and lemon

Lunch- roasted fish and tomatoes

Dinner- 1 beef steak and salad

Day 6

Breakfast- one cup of unsweetened coffee

Lunch- 200gr of chicken and a salad

Dinner- 2 hard-boiled eggs and grated carrots

Day 7

Breakfast- unsweetened coffee

Lunch- a piece of meat and some fruit

Dinner- by choice

Note: While on this diet, you should not consume alcohol, sugar products or salt.

The meat can be roasted, fried, boiled, or braised.

5. Lose a Stone on the Fruitarian Diet

Have you heard of the Fruitarian diet? It is a diet that consists of eating mostly fruit, which I have done, but I have added protein to the diet to make it healthier.

I normally like eating fruit right up to dinner time, so I decided I would just eat protein with salad at mealtimes. Sometimes with carrots. It's something that I have been doing since I started the Chemical Diet here.

The Fruitarian diet is not a practical diet that should be followed for a long time. I would say do it for one week and then wean yourself back onto other foods for the next three weeks before starting the diet again. Just like the Chemical Diet (which I have written about here). I do the Chemical Diet for one week, then I eat fruit and combine it with protein, vegetables, and salad for my evening meals.

The following food plan for the Fruitarian diet should only be followed for one week if you are just going to stick to eating fruit only, which I could not do myself. Some people just eat fruit all week long, but I personally would not try this, so I eat fruits along with having a protein evening meal like fish with salad, beef steak, and vegetables or chicken.

Here is the food plan:

Eat any of these foods for one week:

Breakfast	Large avocado with
	½ tbsp freshly
	ground linseeds
	Large slice melon
	25g hazelnuts + 25g raw
	sunflower seeds
	500ml freshly grapefruit juice
Mid-morning	Large handful mixed raw nuts &
	seeds
	2 apples or pears or peaches
	1 banana
	3 slices of melon

Lunch	Nut & seed mix: 25g walnuts
	+ 10-15 Brazil nuts +
	25g pine nuts
	8-10 raw olives
	¼ cucumber, sliced
	2-3 raw tomatoes
	Juice of 3-4 lemons
Mid-afternoon	Large handful cashew nuts
	2 apples/pears/peaches
	500ml freshly squeezed
	melon juice
	8-10 raw olives
Evening Meal	¼ cucumber, sliced
	2-3 raw tomatoes

Fish

or 2 Eggs

or Beef steak

or chicken breast

or tuna

salad ie celery and lettuce

carrots

Bowlful fresh berries

(vary choice)

Juice of 3-4 lemons

Eat any of these foods throughout the week. The meal plan is just an idea of how you can diet using fruit and combining it with protein and healthy foods. One thing I do not do is eat fruit late at night!

6. Lose a Stone Using the Coffee Diet

If you want to lose more than a stone then try this **incredible diet.** It has worked for many people who are desperate to lose pounds including myself.

It is, also, similar to the Chemical Diet.

This diet is a great detox too.

See the next page for the full diet plan.

Day 1

Breakfast- one cup of unsweetened coffee

Lunch- 2 hard-boiled eggs

Dinner- a piece of meat and lemon-based salad

Day 2

Breakfast- one cup of unsweetened coffee and

a piece of wholemeal toast dry

Lunch- 2 hard-boiled eggs

Dinner- a piece of ham, salad and one cup of

sour cream

Day 3

Breakfast- one cup of unsweetened coffee

Lunch- vegetable and fruit mix

Dinner- 2 hard-boiled eggs, a piece of ham and

salad

Day 4

Breakfast- one cup of unsweetened coffee

Lunch- 2 hard-boiled eggs and carrot juice

Dinner- a piece of meat and lemon-based salad

Day 5

Breakfast- grated carrots and lemon

Lunch- roasted fish and tomatoes

Dinner- 1 beef steak and salad

Day 6

Breakfast- one cup of unsweetened coffee

Lunch- 200gr of chicken and a salad

Dinner- 2 hard-boiled eggs and grated carrots

Day 7

Breakfast- unsweetened coffee

Lunch- a piece of meat and some fruit

Dinner- by choice

Note: While on this diet, you should not consume alcohol, sugar or salt. The meat can be roasted, fried, boiled, or braised.

7. Six High-Protein Foods to Eat With Eggs

for Faster Weight Loss

Did you know there are five high-protein foods that are better than eating eggs?

Apparently, if you eat certain foods with eggs, they will pack even more protein. In this post, I have listed some surprising foods that have more protein than eggs.

Find out more...

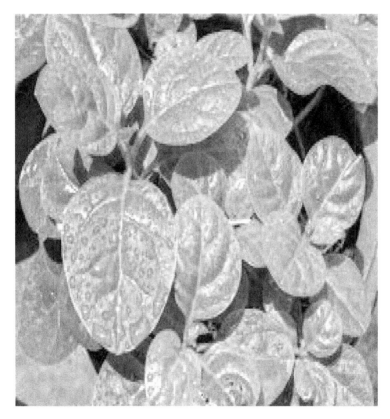

I eat these foods all the time.

1. **Spinach**

Spinach is a good source of iron, and calcium and has a lot of protein. It has rich plant-based omega-3 fatty acids and folate, which can reduce the risk of heart disease, stroke, and osteoporosis.

Use spinach with salads and add it to either your omelette or scrambled eggs. Keep eating this recipe for a few days for weight loss.

2. **Dried Tomatoes**

Tomatoes are packed with the antioxidant lycopene, which studies show can decrease your risk of bladder, lung, prostate, skin, and stomach cancers and reduce the risk of coronary artery disease.

Eat tomatoes with salads and add them to your omelette.

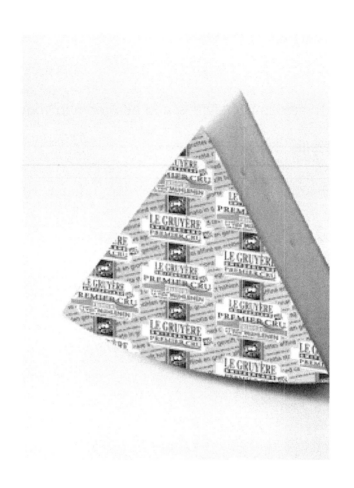

Photo credit: en.wikimedia.org

3. Gruyere Cheese

Gruyere cheese is Swiss cheese. It contains

49

30% more protein than an egg in one slice.

Eat this cheese with eggs and spinach.

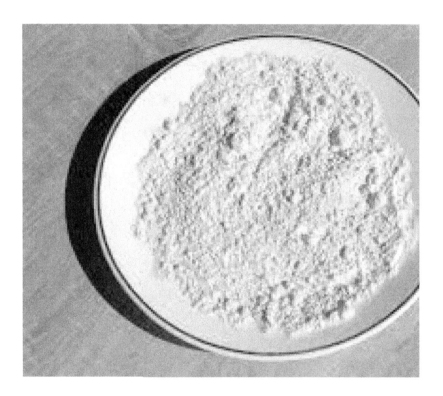

Photo credit: en.wikipedia.org

4. Chickpea Flour

Chickpea flour is high in iron, magnesium, potassium, and fibre. Use it to cook all kinds of recipes for a healthy meal. For instance, use it when cooking omelettes, french toast, crepes, and pancakes. I have used Chickpea flour when cooking omelettes and it comes out tastier than without it.

5. Pumpkin Seeds

Pumpkin seeds are crunchy and are a winner. One cup contains twice as much protein as an egg. They are high in iron, potassium, phosphorus, magnesium, and zinc.

Add pumpkin seeds to salads, and yogurt, or eat them as a snack on their own. They are delicious. I always eat them as a snack.

6. Kamut

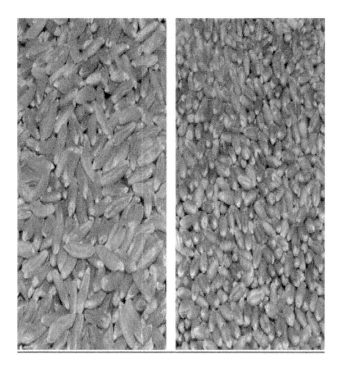

Photo credit: commons.wikimedia.org

Kamut is an ancient grain. It has a lot of protein. It's high in magnesium, potassium, and iron in one cup. Eating Kamut can reduce cholesterol, blood sugar, and inflammation in the body.

You can eat Kamut with salads or on its own. I eat it with salad and eggs.

8. Five Drinks to Help You Lose Weight

Do you want to lose weight? I have heard how some drinks can benefit us in losing weight.

I came across this video by chance when I was searching on Youtube, so I thought I would share it here.

I have also found an article that will tell you how this can work.

Read on and watch the video to learn more.

The Best 5 Healthy Weight Loss Drinks That

Work will tell you how this can work.

Here are the 5 drinks that will work.

1. Water

2. Green Tea

3. Vegetable Smoothie

4. Coffee

5. Skinny Yogurt

Watch the video and start learning how these

drinks can help you with your weight loss.

https://www.youtube.com/watch?v=Q_uiHQfUpi

s

9. Drinking Oolong Tea for Weight Loss

Did you know that if you drink Oolong tea it can help you lose weight? Have you tried it?

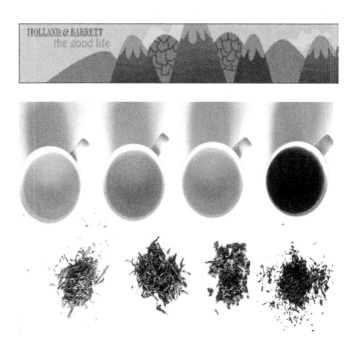

Photo credit: en.wikipedia.org

I have been drinking Oolong tea and it has curbed my bad eating habits along with boosting my metabolism. I am also doing the Chemical Diet this week so drinking Oolong tea has helped me not to crave food.

Oolong tea is made from the leaves, buds and stems of the *Camellia sinensis* plant. Oolong tea is slightly fermented and semi-oxidized, giving it a taste in between black and green teas. The best Oolong tea comes from the Fujian province of China.

Oolong tea is known to provide robust health benefits when consumed regularly. It is packed with antioxidants. Oolong leaf is combined with catechin and caffeine which fight free radicals.

Where Can You Buy Oolong Tea?

Oolong is, also, used for its healing properties and can be found in most shops in the United Kingdom, such as Holland _and Barrett_. I bought a pack of Oolong tea made by Birk and Tang in _Holland and Barrett._ You can find Oolong tea on Amazon.co.uk where you will find plenty of shops selling this tea.

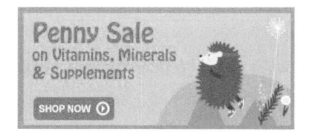

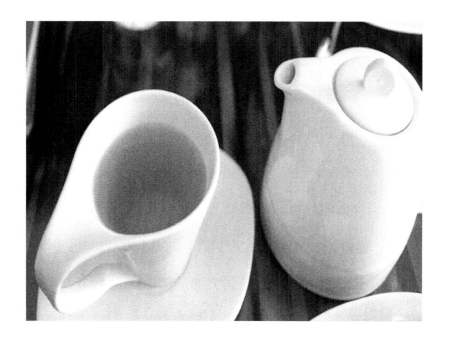

Photo credit: Pixaby

Oolong tea can help with the following things:

1. Boosts your metabolism, which causes weight loss. Drink a cup of Oolong tea in the morning when you wake up, before lunch, and

before dinner. Although, I drink much more than that throughout the day. I have drunk it daily for a week now. It is definitely working for me and I have already lost 4 pounds. You can buy other strains of Oolong tea which may have a stronger taste to it.

2. Lowers Cholesterol and promotes heart health. Oolong tea is semi-oxidized, which produces polyphenol molecules. This helps to dissolve body fat.

3. Increases mental alertness because it contains caffeine.

4. Aids digestion in reducing inflammation for those who suffer from acid reflux and ulcer problems.

5. Promotes healthy hair due to having many

antioxidants in Oolong tea.

6. Gives you healthy looking skin.

7. Stabilises blood sugar if you have type 2 diabetes.

8. Prevents tooth decay.

9. Prevents osteoporosis and gives you strong bones.

10. Oolong tea strengthens the immune system. Drinking it can prevent cancer.

How Much Oolong Tea Should You Drink for Significant Weight Loss?

When I drink Oolong tea I steep the tea bag in not-so-hot boiling water and leave it for 5 minutes. Sometimes I just drink the tea with the tea bag still in it.

You are supposed to have 4 cups of Oolong tea per day according to what I have read, but I have drunk at least 6 cups in one day and it made me feel great. I did feel a little tea drunk occasionally when I drank too much of it, but that's if you consume more than 3 cups very quickly.

So, if you like the sound of Oolong tea and you need to lose weight, then buy some today.

Watch the videos about Oolong tea. https://www.youtube.com/watch?v=a692qvemwV0 https://www.youtube.com/watch?v=RGQhiLIT-Fk https://www.youtube.com/watch?v=VMUmWnb

<u>2ZL0</u>

10. Drinking Rooibos Tea for Healthy Slim Life

Have you tried Rooibos tea?

It's a sweet herbal tea that will benefit your health and encourage weight loss.

I bought this tea just recently and have been drinking it daily for 2 weeks now. It has definitely made a difference for me and it has helped me burn fat now that I am losing weight.

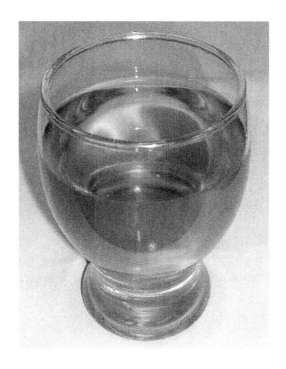

Photo credit: en.wikipedia.org - Rooibos Tea

Here are a few things to consider about why you should drink Rooibos tea:

1. Lots of Antioxidants in Rooibos Tea

The antioxidants in Rooibos tea are good for

your health and if you are trying to lose weight then this tea will benefit you greatly by drinking 3 cups of it throughout the day.

2. No Caffeine in Rooibos Tea

You will never get that caffeine-jittery feeling ever again if you drink this tea.

3. It is Good for Your Skin

Drinking Rooibos tea will help keep your skin clear and smooth. You can apply the powder from the tea bag directly to your bad skin/face or just simply drink the tea. It can improve eczema, sunburn, rashes, dry skin, and irritation.

4. It Helps with Weight Loss

The reason why Rooibos tea is so good at helping you lose weight is that it contains catechins, which have been said to burn fat.

5. Drinking Rooibos Tea will Calm an Upset Stomach

This tea can definitely heal your upset stomach. Just one cup will relieve an upset stomach and reduce inflammation along with bloating.

6. Good for the Heart

Drinking Rooibos tea can improve cardiovascular mortality but it is still unknown why this happens from drinking this tea.

7. Good for Diabetes

Drinking Rooibos tea is good for diabetes,

because it contains aspalathin, which means glucose uptake can be increased, improving its tolerance in just 5 weeks according to a study conducted by the Tokyo University of Agriculture and Technology.

8. Good for the Liver

The antioxidants found in Rooibos tea can protect your liver against damage. It has been shown to reverse some initial damage that may have been caused to the liver and the tea can help to repair it even further.

9. Rooibos Tea Can Prevent Cancer

The tea cannot, sadly, take away cancer that is already there, but it can prevent cancer if the tea is drunk regularly.

10. Helps You to Sleep

If you need a good night's sleep, then drinking Rooibos tea before bedtime can promote a good night's rest. Instead of drinking coffee late at night why not switch to Rooibos tea.

Where Can You Buy Rooibos Tea?

Rooibos tea can be bought in Holland and Barrett shops or online all over the United Kingdom. It is also sold on Amazon sites.

Here are a few video links about Rooibos tea:

https://www.youtube.com/watch?v=Z4oQlq_o GVs

https://www.youtube.com/watch?v=Zl_4xprvi
Kk

https://www.youtube.com/watch?v=MA-
QFOYSnK8

https://www.youtube.com/watch?v=Y4BnHko
mD-s

11. The Egg Fast Diet for Fast Weight Loss

Can you just eat eggs for 3 or 4 days without any other foods?

I have found out that eating eggs alone can help you lose a considerable amount of weight in a week.

The Egg Fast Diet is for fast weight loss alone. Eat 2 eggs for breakfast, lunch and dinner. Only do it for 3 or 4 days and then add salad and other foods either on the fourth or fifth day. Do this every week and see the weight fall off you, but beware, if you suffer from high cholesterol, then this might not be a good idea.

Read how you can **transition from the egg fast diet back** to a healthy diet each week. It's hard going, but it does work.

The **Ketogenic Woman blog** will give you a food plan for the Egg Fast Diet.

I am not sure if this is a healthy thing to do, but I gave it a go, because I really needed to lose a lot of weight for a wedding that I was about to attend. I wanted to buy a decent dress that I would look good in. So, I did the Egg Fast Diet for four days. I definitely lost weight doing it, but I felt so sick by the end of it of eggs that I was relieved to eat other foods. I did lose 11 lbs, which was a huge bonus for me and I felt a surge of energy that I hadn't felt before whilst dieting.

So, if you are interested, I have provided the exact diet plan.

Here is the Egg Fast Diet Plan below:

Meal 1: Coffee with Sweet Leaf stevia

Meal 2: 2 eggs scrambled or fried in 1 tbsp butter

Meal 3: 3 hard-boiled eggs mashed with 2 tbsp mayonnaise

Snack: 2 oz hard cheese (any kind)

Meal 4: omelette made with 2 eggs and 1 or 2 oz cheese

Snack only if hungry (1 or 2 oz cheese)

Total for the day: 7 eggs, 7 tbsp fat (2 mayo), 6 oz cheese but usually only 4 or 5.

If you don't like eggs then this is not the diet for you. Only do this diet for 4 days and no more.

Another great diet that can help you lose up to one stone in a week is the Chemical Diet which I have talked about in this book.

A video from a Doctor about just eating eggs: https://www.youtube.com/watch?v=_tdFdPpWK3Q

Watch a video of a guy who did the egg diet : https://www.youtube.com/watch?v=SLsEql31jEQ

The health benefits of eggs:

https://www.youtube.com/watch?v=rdbSy3YKlz

o

Watch the following video about the Egg Fast

Diet:

https://www.youtube.com/watch?v=Wu1bSYm-

uak

Watch another video about a diet called The

Chemical Diet. **It is a one-week diet where**

you can lose one stone.

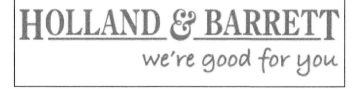

12. How Much Weight Can You Lose in Two Days?

I have a wedding to go to on Friday of this week and I am desperate to lose weight. I have a dress that I want to wear, but I know it's going to be tight on me. Have you ever been in this situation before? Have you ever wanted to get into a dress so badly, but there were only two days left until the wedding? Well, I have come up with a diet that can help with this problem. Check it out below.

So, for the next two days, I am going to eat a lot less. You may wonder how I am going to do this, but I have read how you can lose at least half a stone eating less in a healthy way for two days and then eating normally the rest of the time.

So, I am going to fast for two days and see what happens. I will still eat food, but less food.

Here is my fast diet plan for the next two days.
Eggs will be part of my diet.

You MUST only eat/drink what is on this list for
it to work

Breakfast:

1 soft or hard-boiled egg

1 mug of oolong tea (Chinese tea no sugar
added or sweetener)

Lunch:

2 hard-boiled eggs

1 mug of oolong tea - no sugar or sweetener

Dinner:

1 fresh fish grilled or tin of tuna in springwater
or 1 grilled steak 127 calories,

served with some lettuce and cucumber - NO seasoning

1 mug of Oolong tea - no sugar or sweetener

Before Bed: 1 mug of Oolong tea - no sugar or sweetener

You can drink Green tea instead of Oolong tea if you prefer or ordinary breakfast tea but do not use milk - Stevia sweeteners aloud. Coffee is allowed but without milk or sugar - or use Stevia sweeteners.

You can buy Chinese Oolong tea on Amazon or at Holland and Barrett.

VERY IMPORTANT:

You must also drink a glass of water when you wake up (before breakfast), another between breakfast and lunch, another before lunch, another between lunch and dinner, another before dinner, another within an hour or two after dinner, and one more before bed. Put nothing in your water.

I did this for two days and I lost a total of six pounds in weight. So, it can work. I didn't eat grilled steak, just fish for both of those days, so doing this may be better for weight loss. I didn't put the weight back on even though I drank some wine. I continued with the diet for another three days the following week. After three days I ate sensibly but did not have more than 1500 calories. I continued to lose weight easily using

Read more about diets that I have talked about on Skinny is Best website here https://www.skinnyisbest.co.uk/

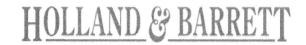

Buy Oolong tea here

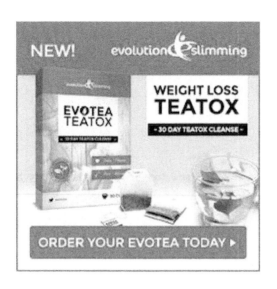

13. The Atkins Diet

Have you tried the Atkins Diet? It's a diet that's been around for a long time. It's a diet that can help you to lose pounds quite quickly.

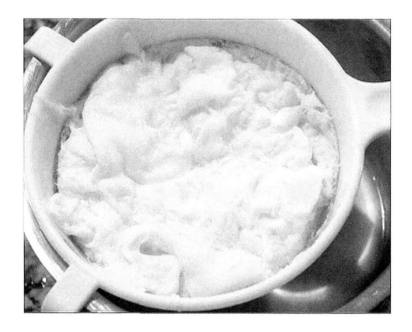

Eggs are protein and can be eaten on the Atkins Diet - eat as many of them as you like!

From what I understand, the Atkins Diet can put glucose levels down. I couldn't believe this at first, so I gave it a go because my doctor told me that I was pre-diabetic. I stopped eating bad carbohydrates and now I have been told by my doctor that my glucose levels have gone down. Doing the Atkins Diet can help you if you think you might be pre-diabetic or if you are diabetic. Give it a go because it will work!

Phase 1 of the Atkins diet tells you to only have up to 20 grams of carbohydrates per day.

Phase 2 of the Atkins diet tells you to only have

up to 40 grams of carbohydrates per day.

Check out the Atkins Diet online here.

I have done this diet a few times in the past and it has always helped me to lose weight. Give it a go and see where it will get you.

Watch the following videos:

https://www.youtube.com/watch?v=cuqR5VxnDUM

https://www.youtube.com/watch?v=PN0YLnjViU8

14. Lose Weight on the Lemon Drink Diet

Do you think you could be motivated to lose 10 pounds in a week? Well, I know I would be.

Here is a diet that I have found, where you can lose 10 pounds. All you have to do is stick to it. So, can you do that?

I gave it a try. It was my first new year diet that I experimented with. So, here it is:

Breakfast:

Start your day off with a Lemon drink - one glass of mild water and 3 tablespoons of fresh lemon juice (squeezed from lemons)

Lemon water will hydrate and alkalise your body when drunk in the morning. The drink will cleanse your liver of all toxins and activate your metabolism.

After half an hour, eat either two apples or two oranges, or one grapefruit. If fruit is not enough and you are still hungry, then you can have half a cup of nuts, almonds, or hazelnuts.

The combination of fruit and nuts will provide you with nutrients and healthy fats for the whole day. Your stomach will feel full and satisfied.

Lunch:

Eat pure protein. Eat either 5 ounces of skinless chicken or veal, or fresh fish.

Add 1 container of Greek yogurt

Snack can be a banana or green salad with no

extra dressings

Dinner:

Dinner should be before 6 pm and after that, you should not eat anything. After this time you should give your digestive system a rest. You can only have water or tea after 6 pm.

Dinner should be:

Two hard-boiled eggs

Green salad with slices

of cucumber, extra-virgin olive oil

Himalayan salt allowed but just a little.

After dinner, you can have a few cups of Green tea, but sometimes I have Oolong tea. If you have at least 3 cups of Green tea you will burn at least 80 calories. I will be having about 5 cups before I go to bed to see how that works out.

If you stick to this diet, I guarantee you will lose at least 10 pounds after seven days.

15. The Dukan Diet -

The Attack Phase is Worth Doing

The Dukan Diet plan is a French diet and was designed by Dr. Pierre Dukan who wrote a book about it. I have, in the past, followed this diet and in 11 days I lost a total of 12 pounds.

Anyone can do this diet plan. It was easy and I still lost more weight every day after those 11 days.

Here is what I did during my first 10 days on the Dukan Diet.

My First Ten Days on Attack Phase

The first phase is called Attack Phase on the Dukan Diet where you just eat pure protein and oat bran every day. You can start the plan off by doing 3 days, 5 days or even 10 days if you need to lose a lot of weight in the Attack Phase. You can lose a good amount of weight on this first phase, so if you do have a lot to lose, then do 10 days on this plan. I did 10 days and I did not feel hungry at all whilst on it. The oat bran that you eat every morning consists of one and half tablespoons, which you are supposed to have each day on the Dukan Diet.

I have added a list of foods and drinks that you can have during this phase below if you want to get started straight away.

Food and Drinks

During the Attack Phase you can only eat pure protein foods and have one and half tablespoons of oat bran for breakfast or any time of the day. You can make a pancake using the oat bran, which I did myself each day (see below for the recipe).

Here are the foods and drinks that are allowed on Attack Phase:

Skinless Fish

Sardines in tomato sauce or brine

Oat bran – 1 1/2 tablespoons per day only

Tuna

Skinless chicken (no wings or chicken with crumbs)

Steak

Onions can be used when cooking, i.e. cooked on a pan with meat or in the oven.

Sweetener - Splenda (except fructose-based), vinegars, mustard, spices, herbs, garlic, lemon juice (as a spice), sugar-free natural tomato ketchup (in moderation), sugar-free chewing gum.

Fat-free Greek yogurt

Fat-free vanilla yogurt (such as Onken vanilla yogurt - do not eat fruit yogurt containing bits of fruit it can ruin the diet)

Eggs

Prawns, mussels or any seafood

Ham (low fat and lean)

Lean beef, veal, and rabbit mince but avoid ribs

Beef and veal

Sugar-free jelly

Fat-free cottage cheese

Tea and coffee and at least 2 litres of water per day

Chicken liver

Diet coke and skimmed milk

Oat Bran Pancake Recipe

Contents:

1 1/2 tablespoons of oat bran

1 egg

2 tablespoons of fat-free Greek yogurt or fat-

free vanilla yogurt

Splenda (for a sweetening taste)

Cooking Method:

Mix the contents and fry on a pan where you will see it turn into a sweet tasting pancake. If you prefer it not to be sweet, then just add lemon, pepper, and garlic for the taste to the contents then cook in a frying pan. Spray the pan lightly with oil. I have eaten this pancake most mornings for breakfast.

The Next Phase - Cruise Phase

This next part of the diet is where you can add vegetables and salad. This phase is alternated each day, so the first day is on pure protein (PP) and then the next day you have protein and vegetables (PV). This continues like this until you get down to your desired weight.

My Opinion of the Dukan Diet

Whilst I was doing the Attack Phase, I felt very full of what I had eaten. Eating the oat bran each morning gave me energy and fullness to help me succeed further in the diet. I lost 12 pounds during the Attack Phase.

Of course, I had to lose more than that to get to my desired weight.

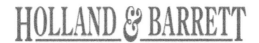

16. The New Updated Dukan Diet

The Dukan Diet's food plan has been recently updated. Now it's a more acceptable diet.

The new eating plan for the diet now adds wholemeal bread, fruit, starchy foods and one celebration meal per week. You will lose weight gradually and healthily on the new plan.

On the new Dukan Diet plan you can eat protein for a minimum of one day or longer (no more than 5 days), then you will add on foods each day for a week and then start with protein for one day again.

100

Previously, the Dukan Diet was much harder to do, but you could succeed to lose a mega amount of pounds in the process. I know this because I did the diet myself and lost a stone in three weeks. Now, the diet is much easier for those who don't want to stick to a strict food plan.

Here is a food plan that you can follow on the new updated Dukan Diet:

Meal Plan:

Monday - Eat protein all day

Tuesday - Eat protein along with vegetables on this day

Wednesday - protein, vegetables and add fruit on this day

Thursday - protein, vegetables, fruit and bread

Friday - protein, vegetables, fruit, bread, and cheese eg. goats cheese

Saturday - protein, vegetables, fruit, bread, cheese, and carbs eg. tandoori chicken with red lentil dhal

Sunday - celebration meal - This is a three-course meal with a small glass of wine

After the first week, you can continue on with the diet as set out in the above meal plan.

So, why not check out Pierre Dukan's new book to see what it's all about:

The Book can be bought at the following link: http://www.amazon.co.uk/The-Dukan-Diet-Dr-

Pierre/dp/1473609941

17. A Fat-Burning Meal Plan

I came across this fat-burning diet, a nutritious meal plan, by chance when I was searching on the internet for a healthy way of dieting.

The following fat-burning diet meal plan looks completely healthy, so I have given it a go and used it to lose a few pounds.

Find out more...

Here is the link for the fat-burning diet meal plan which has 6 weeks of food plans to follow:

A Fat Burning Diet Meal Plan for Six Weeks

The meals are easy to prepare and they will definitely rev up your metabolism helping you to burn fat during this fat burning diet meal plan. All the foods are nutritious, so this will benefit you in the long run.

One of the foods on the meal plan that is said to be the most nutritious and will help your body go into a fat-burning process is Salmon. The Omega-3 fatty acids in this fish can lower bad cholesterol and boost your mood. It will also help to fight those dreaded wrinkles that we get in later life. So, I think I will be eating more Salmon.

Here is the meal plan that I have put together using some of the foods from the above meal plan link above. I have decided that I will eat the following for one week to see how I get on. I will update this article to let you know how I got on.

The following meal plan can be followed all the time as a lifestyle diet.

Monday

Breakfast:

2 Scrambled Eggs

1 large grapefruit

Snack

25 almonds

Lunch:

Turkey in a wrap

1 apple

Snack:

10 grapes

Dinner:

Chicken and a small portion of wholemeal

Pasta, Side salad

Tuesday

Breakfast:

2 Tbsp of peanut butter with 1 piece of

wholemeal toast

1 banana

Snack:

A small bowl of raisins

Lunch:

Tuna and a small portion of wholemeal Pasta

Snack:

0% fat Greek yogurt

Dinner:

Salmon with

2 cups of broccoli

Wednesday

Breakfast:

2 Eggs and Ham

1 large grapefruit

Snack:

25 almonds

Lunch:

Tuna with salad

1 apple

Snack:

1 piece of string cheese

Dinner:

Fish with salad

1 small sweet potato

Thursday

Breakfast:

2 Eggs scrambled

0% fat Greek yogurt

Snack:

2 Tbsp of hummus

Lunch:

Ham salad (tomatoes, cucumber and lettuce)

Snack:

1 banana

Dinner:

Fish and side salad

1 cup of brown rice

2 cups of broccoli

Friday

Breakfast:

0% fat Greek yogurt

1 large grapefruit

Snack:

10 grapes

Lunch:

Salad with ham

25 almonds

Snack:

30 baby carrots

4 Tbsp of hummus

110

Dinner:

Chicken and spinach

1 cup of brown rice

2 cups of snow peas

Saturday

Breakfast:

Loaded Vegetable Omelette

Snack:

1 banana

Lunch:

Turkey Wrap

1 apple

Snack:

10 cherry tomatoes

2 Tbsp of hummus

Dinner:

Lemon Chicken with Rice

2 cups of broccoli

Snack:

1 apple

Sunday

Breakfast:

Loaded Vegetable Omelette

1 banana

Snack:

15 baby carrots, 2 Tbsp of hummus

Lunch:

Eat out day

If you don't eat out for lunch then have the following:

Salmon and salad

1 apple

Snack:

no snack

Dinner:

Small bowl of Chicken with wholemeal pasta (small portion)

1 cup of broccoli

If you want to see Week 2,3,4,5 and 6, then **click here.**

The diet gets better so check out the fat burning meal plan here, for foods to eat as you get into this fat-burning weight loss diet.

I did try this diet but I mostly ate Salmon which I got bored with after a while. I lost 6 pounds even though I only stuck to it for 3 days. So, it's worth trying.

18. The Thirty-Day Crunch Challenge is a Good Way to Start Your Fitness Regime

Has anyone heard of the 30-day crunch challenge? I was given this challenge by a friend who told me about it. Personally, I think it's a great way to start an exercise regime.

The 30-day crunch challenge is to get you motivated into doing exercise, but doing much less exercise than usual.

Why not give it a go!

I have been doing the Chemical Diet so doing the 30-day crunch challenge will be a bonus workout for anyone whilst on this plan. It's a good idea to do something like this if you are just starting out on a diet.

So here it is:

The 30-Day Crunch Challenge

A crunch is like a sit-up, but you do not go all the way up. Lay down on your back and bend your knees. Then lift your head and shoulders slightly upwards and feel your abdomen tighten. Here is how you do the crunch challenge.

Day 1.... 20 crunches

Day 2.... 25 crunches

Day 3.... 30 crunches

Day 4... Rest

Day 5... 40 crunches

Day 6... 45 crunches

Day 7... 50 crunches

Day 8... Rest

Day 9... 60 crunches

Day 10... 65 crunches

Day 11... 70 crunches

Day 12... Rest

Day 13... 80 crunches

Day 14... 90 crunches

Day 15... 95 crunches

Day 16... Rest

Day 17... 100 crunches

Day 18... 105 crunches

Day 19... 110 crunches

Day 20... Rest

Day 21... 115 crunches

Day 22... 120 crunches

Day 23... 125 crunches

Day 24... Rest

Day 25... 130 crunches

Day 26... 135 crunches

Day 27... 140 crunches

Day 28... Rest

Day 29... 145 crunches

Day 30... 150 crunches

The good thing about this challenge is that you can rest from them every 3 days, which is a bonus for me.   So, who will do this challenge? Give it a try!

19. The Thirty-Day Squat Challenge is a Good Way to Start Your Fitness Regime

Has anyone heard of the 30-day squat challenge? It's a similar routine to the crunch challenge.

The 30-day squat challenge is to get you motivated into doing exercise, but doing much less exercise than usual. You can do this 30-day squat challenge if you are on a fast weight loss diet like the Chemical Diet.

The Squat Challenge

A squat is standing and bending your knees with your arms out in front of you as if you are going to sit down. Do this exercise for 30 days along with the crunch challenge. This is how you do it.

Day 1-50 squats

Day 2-55 squats

Day 3-60 squats

Day 4-Rest

Day 5-70 squats

Day 6-75 squats

Day 7-80 squats

Day 8-Rest

Day 9-100 squats

Day 10-105 squats

Day 11-110 squats

Day 12-Rest

Day 13-130 squats

Day 14-135 squats

Day 15- 140 squats

Day 16-Rest

Day 17-150 squats

Day 18- 155 squats

Day 19- 160 squats

Day 20-Rest

Day 21- 180 squats

Day 22- 185 squats

Day 23- 190 squats

Day 24-Rest

Day 25- 220 squats

Day 26- 225 squats

Day 27- 230 squats

Day 28-Rest

Day 29- 240 squats

Day 30- 250 squats

The good thing about this challenge is that you can rest from them every 3 days, which is a bonus for anyone. Give it a try!

Watch the following video about the Chemical Diet: The one-week diet where you can lose one   stone:

https://www.youtube.com/watch?v=oCEwBv

U2Ar0

Watch another video about the 30-day Squat Challenge:

https://www.youtube.com/watch?v=s9Cr-

_ASR0A

20. The 5-4-3-2-1 Workout

I don't know what you have heard about exercise regimes, but I have heard about the 5-4-3-2-1 workout that I greatly recommend for those that cannot do too much exercise.

I am on the Chemical Diet at present and this exercise regime is a bonus workout that can be incorporated whilst doing any kind of diet. Take a look below and start this regime a couple of days before you start your diet. It will boost your energy and help you feel more positive about your diet.

I have been doing the 5-4-3-2-1 workout daily.

It's definitely the best exercise regime I have adopted in a long time. Please give it a try.

Here is the workout exercise regime that I want to share with you.

The 5-4-3-2-1 Workout

5 minutes: Cardio - do anything you want: walk, run, jump rope, elliptical, bike

- at home

  - 1 minute high knees

  - 1 minute jumping jacks

  - 1 minute front kicks

  - 1 minute run in place

4 minutes

- 1 minute lunges or walking lunges

- 1 minute mountain climbers

- repeat for 4 minutes

3 minutes

- 10 push-ups/rest

- 15 triceps dips/rest

- repeat for 3 minutes

2 minutes

- 30 seconds regular squats

- 30 seconds jump squats

- 30 seconds regular squats

- 30 seconds jump squats

1 minute

- plank

The workout should take about 15 minutes;

intermediate repeat for a total of 2 times through; advanced repeat for a total of 3 times through.

Drink water and take breaks when you need them. If you are just starting out, take more breaks, especially between each section.

21. Intermittent Fasting For a Healthy Lifestyle

Intermittent fasting (IF) is a dietary pattern that involves alternating periods of fasting and eating. It is not a specific diet but rather an eating pattern. The idea is to restrict the time during which you eat, typically by skipping breakfast and eating your first meal later in the day, and finishing your last meal earlier in the evening.

There are different ways to practice IF, but the most common ones are:

- Time-restricted feeding: This involves fasting for a certain number of hours each day, usually between 12 and 16

129

hours. For example, you might eat all of your meals within an 8-hour window (e.g., noon to 8 pm) and fast for the remaining 16 hours.

- Alternate day fasting: This involves eating normally one day and then restricting calories to 500-600 the next day.

- 5:2 diet: This involves eating normally for five days of the week and then restricting calories to 500-600 for two non-consecutive days of the week.

Intermittent fasting has been shown to have several health benefits, including weight loss, improved metabolic health, and reduced inflammation. However, it may not be suitable for everyone, especially those with a history of disordered eating or certain medical conditions. It's important to speak with a healthcare provider before starting any new diet or eating pattern.

Can you lose weight using intermittent fasting?

Yes, intermittent fasting can be an effective way to lose weight. By reducing the amount of time you spend eating and creating a calorie deficit, your body is forced to burn stored fat for energy, which can result in weight loss.

Research has shown that intermittent fasting can be as effective as traditional calorie-restricted diets for weight loss, and it may have some advantages over other diets. For example, some people find it easier to stick to an intermittent fasting regimen because they don't have to worry about counting calories or restricting certain foods.

It's important to note, however, that weight loss is not guaranteed with intermittent fasting. It's still possible to overeat during the periods when you're allowed to eat, which could offset the calorie deficit created by the fasting period. Additionally, individual results may vary depending on factors such as age, sex, starting weight, and overall health.

As with any weight loss plan, it's important to talk to a healthcare provider before starting intermittent fasting to make sure it's a safe and

appropriate choice for you.

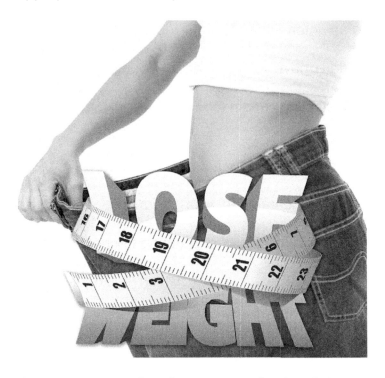

Can you use fat from your body doing

intermittent fasting no matter what you eat?

Intermittent fasting can help you lose fat by

creating a calorie deficit, which means that

133

you're burning more calories than you're consuming. However, it's important to note that what you eat during your eating periods can also have an impact on your weight loss results.

If you eat a lot of high-calorie, high-fat foods during your eating periods, you may not see the same weight loss results as if you were eating a healthy, balanced diet. Additionally, if you consume more calories than your body needs during your eating periods, you may not lose weight at all, even if you're fasting.

To optimize fat loss during intermittent fasting, it's important to focus on eating nutrient-dense, whole foods during your eating periods, such as lean protein, vegetables, fruits, and whole grains. This can help you feel fuller and more satisfied with fewer calories, making it easier to maintain a calorie deficit.

It's also important to pay attention to portion sizes and limit your intake of processed and high-calorie foods, which can quickly add up and derail your weight loss efforts.

Overall, while intermittent fasting can be an effective way to lose fat, what you eat during your eating periods is also important for optimizing your results.

Is intermittent fasting healthy for everyone?

Intermittent fasting may not be healthy for everyone, particularly for those who are underweight, pregnant or breastfeeding, have a history of disordered eating, or have certain medical conditions.

People with a history of disordered eating, such as anorexia or bulimia, should avoid intermittent fasting because it may trigger unhealthy behaviors around food and body image.

Individuals who are underweight or have a history of malnutrition may not have sufficient energy stores to safely practice intermittent fasting and may require additional nutrition and medical supervision.

Pregnant and breastfeeding women need additional nutrients and calories to support the growth and development of their babies, so it's not recommended for them to practice intermittent fasting.

People with certain medical conditions, such as diabetes, low blood sugar, and kidney disease, may need to monitor their blood sugar levels closely during periods of fasting and should consult with their healthcare provider before starting an intermittent fasting regimen.

Overall, it's important to talk to a healthcare provider before starting any new diet or eating pattern to ensure that it's safe and appropriate for your individual needs and medical history.

How does autophagy work whilst doing

intermittent fasting?

Autophagy is a natural process in which cells break down and recycle damaged or dysfunctional parts of themselves to maintain cellular health. It is triggered when the body is under stress, such as during periods of fasting.

During intermittent fasting, the body switches from using glucose for energy to using stored fat for energy. This leads to a decrease in insulin levels, which is thought to be a trigger for autophagy. In addition, the decreased availability of glucose and amino acids during fasting may also stimulate autophagy.

Autophagy helps to clear out damaged or misfolded proteins, excess lipids, and other cellular debris that can accumulate over time and contribute to various diseases, including cancer, Alzheimer's, and Parkinson's.

While intermittent fasting has been shown to increase autophagy in animal studies, the evidence in humans is limited and conflicting. Some studies have shown an increase in autophagy markers in response to intermittent fasting, while others have not.

It's important to note that while autophagy has potential health benefits, more research is needed to fully understand its effects on health and disease. It's also not clear how much fasting is needed to trigger autophagy or if other factors, such as exercise or sleep, may also influence the process.

Can intermittent fasting get rid of cancer?

There is currently no scientific evidence to support the claim that intermittent fasting can cure cancer. While some studies have suggested that fasting may have potential health benefits and may help to prevent cancer, it is not a substitute for conventional cancer treatment.

Cancer is a complex disease that requires individualized treatment based on the type and stage of cancer, as well as the patient's overall health. Conventional cancer treatments, such as chemotherapy, radiation, and surgery, have been shown to be effective in many cases and are recommended by healthcare professionals.

While some studies have suggested that fasting may have potential health benefits and may help to prevent cancer, it is important to note that these studies are limited and more research is needed to fully understand the relationship between fasting and cancer prevention.

It's also important to talk to a healthcare provider before starting any new diet or fasting regimen, especially if you have cancer or are undergoing cancer treatment, as fasting may not be safe or appropriate for all individuals.

Are there any cases to suggest that intermittent fasting has cured cancer patients?

To date, there is no scientific evidence to support the claim that intermittent fasting can cure cancer. While there are some studies that suggest that fasting may have potential health benefits and may help to prevent cancer, there is no reliable evidence that intermittent fasting can cure cancer or replace conventional cancer treatments.

It's important to remember that cancer is a complex disease that requires individualized treatment based on the type and stage of cancer, as well as the patient's overall health.

Conventional cancer treatments, such as chemotherapy, radiation, and surgery, have been shown to be effective in many cases and are recommended by healthcare professionals.

While some cancer patients may choose to incorporate fasting or other dietary interventions into their treatment plan, it's important to do so under the guidance of a healthcare provider and as a complementary approach to conventional cancer treatment, not as a replacement for it.

It's also important to be cautious of anecdotal reports or individual cases that suggest that fasting has cured cancer, as these are not supported by scientific evidence and may be misleading or even dangerous.

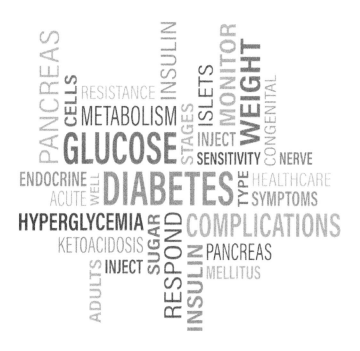

Is there any research to support intermittent fasting?

Yes, there is a growing body of scientific research that supports the potential health benefits of intermittent fasting. Many studies have shown that intermittent fasting may help to improve various markers of health, such as blood sugar control, cholesterol levels, and inflammation.

Some of the potential health benefits of intermittent fasting supported by scientific research include:

- Weight loss: Intermittent fasting can lead to reduced calorie intake, which can lead to weight loss over time.
- Improved blood sugar control: Intermittent fasting has been shown to improve insulin sensitivity and lower blood sugar levels, which may reduce

the risk of type 2 diabetes.

- Lowered inflammation: Intermittent fasting has been shown to reduce inflammation in the body, which may have a variety of health benefits.

- Improved heart health: Intermittent fasting may help to improve cholesterol levels, blood pressure, and other markers of heart health.

- Brain function: Some studies have suggested that intermittent fasting may have cognitive benefits, such as improved memory and concentration.

It's important to note that while intermittent fasting has potential health benefits, it may not be suitable for everyone. People who are underweight, pregnant or breastfeeding, have a history of disordered eating or have certain medical conditions should talk to a healthcare provider before starting an intermittent fasting regimen.

Conclusion

In conclusion, intermittent fasting has gained significant attention in recent years due to its potential health benefits. While more research is needed to fully understand the effects of intermittent fasting on different populations and health conditions, existing studies suggest that it may help with weight loss, blood sugar regulation, and inflammation reduction.

It is important to note that intermittent fasting

may not be suitable for everyone, especially individuals with certain health conditions or who are pregnant or breastfeeding. It is recommended to consult with a healthcare professional before starting an intermittent fasting regimen.

Furthermore, it is essential to follow a balanced and nutritious diet during the feeding periods and to avoid overeating to reap the benefits of intermittent fasting fully. Additionally, combining intermittent fasting with regular exercise can enhance its effects on overall health.

In summary, intermittent fasting may be a useful tool for those looking to improve their health and manage their weight. However, it is important to approach it safely and with caution and to consult with a healthcare professional before starting any new diet or exercise regimen.

The Conclusion of this Book

So, that's it! I hope you enjoyed reading this book. Please leave a review if you enjoyed reading it and if it was helpful for you.

Thank you so much for reading.

Check out the website for lots more diet plans and information:

Skinny is Best - https://www.skinnyisbest.co.uk/